T0266001

Is Community Rating Essential to Managed Competition?

Mark A. Hall

The AEI Press

Publisher for the American Enterprise Institute

WASHINGTON, D.C.

1994

. To order call toll free 1-800-462-6420 or 1-717-794-3800. For all other inquiries please contact the AEI Press, 1150 Seventeenth Street, N.W., Washington, D.C. 20036 or call 1-800-862-5801.

ISBN 978-0-8447-7018-5
ISBN 0-8447-7018-3

The AEI Press
Publisher for the American Enterprise Institute
1150 17th Street, N.W., Washington, D.C. 20036

Contents

Perhaps the most overlooked aspect of the health care reform debate so far is whether health insurance should be community-rated in a system of managed competition. A move toward community rating is generally considered desirable,[1] yet fundamental differences exist among the proposals now pending before Congress—differences that reflect underlying disagreements over the basic philosophy of how health care markets should work and how best to spread the social burden of universal access. The Clinton administration, for instance, has not been bashful in admitting that one goal of requiring large employers to participate in health alliances is that, as a consequence of community rating, large alliances ensure a much broader base over which to spread the higher costs of enrolling Medicaid recipients. Because these and other public policy implications of community rating have yet to be rigorously explored, this essay will describe how various forms of community rating work and will analyze their fairness, efficiency, and feasibility. Finding strong arguments on both sides of the debate, the essay concludes that neither pure community rating nor unconstrained risk rating should prevail. Instead, a variety of compromise rating and risk-adjustment systems should be considered.

The Forms of Community Rating

The term "community rating" has been used to describe an array of pricing mechanisms. In essence, these various mechanisms work to compress the range of variation in individual premiums produced by experience rating. Three forms of rate compression have been proposed: strict (or pure) community rating, adjusted community rating (or community rating by class), and rating bands. The result under any of these is that, while the average cost of insurance is not affected, the spread between the high and the low ends is greatly reduced. The extent to which a market-based reform can employ community rating is independent of the

---

Derrick Max, a research assistant at the American Enterprise Institute, provided many valuable insights that refined my analysis of a number of crucial points.

type of market reform pursued, so long as the reform mandates universal coverage. Either community rating or experience rating is compatible with both purchasing cooperatives and medical savings accounts, under either an individual or an employer mandate. More critical to community-rating compatibility is whether market reforms call for voluntary or mandatory purchase. My focus is on mandatory purchase.

President Clinton's plan calls for strict community rating within each regional and corporate alliance, meaning that insurers may not vary their premiums to any degree according to age, gender, health status, or occupational category. Strict community rating allows premiums to vary only according to geographic location, level and type of benefits (for example, HMO versus fee-for-service), and family status. Therefore, each health plan's price must reflect the average costs to its community of subscribers for each type of policy in each location. This is also the form of community rating recently enacted in New York for individual and small-group purchasers, and it is being phased in by several other states.

Adjusted community rating allows additional variation according to defined demographic classes, usually age and gender. Typically, insurers will form rating categories for male and female groupings in five-year increments. This is the form of community rating used by Blue Cross plans that still offer open enrollment, and it is the form that prevailed in the small-group market before the mid-1980s, when cost pressures caused its disintegration. Senator Don Nickles's bill calls for full age-adjusted community rating, whereas Senator John Chafee's and Representative Jim Cooper's bills allow only a twofold variation based on age.

Rating bands are the least demanding means to accomplish rate compression. Rating bands allow an additional measure of rate variation beyond age-and-gender-adjusted community rating, a measure that reflects to some extent individual health risk associated with prior claims experience or with occupational and industry classifications.[2] The most prominent source of rating-band proposals is the National Association of Insurance Commissioners (NAIC), whose model law draws heavily from the Health Insurance Association of America's proposal for small-group market reform. This reform package, which has been enacted in some fashion in about forty states, requires insurers to limit their premium variation to + or - 25 percent of the average for each demographic grouping within a block of business. Unlimited variation is allowed, however, across age groups. Similar proposals exist in legislation that was considered in the 102d Congress (for example, Representative Dan Rostenkowski's and Senator Lloyd Bentsen's bills). A similar proposal is also contained in Representative Robert Michel's bill now pending, although some of these bills allow less variation than the NAIC's model, or phase down the degree of allowable variation.

In short, most reform proposals that continue to rely on the market for private health insurance require some limitation on the extent to which insurance premiums may reflect individual health risk, but none require insurers to be completely blind to risk. Even strict community rating allows insurers to adjust for location, type and scope of coverage, and family status. There are vast differences, however, in the degree of risk rating allowed by competing proposals. These differences raise public policy issues that go to the fairness, the efficiency, and the feasibility of community rating. I will analyze many dimensions of each of these issues to understand better the complexity of the debate. I conclude that, although pure community rating should be rejected, one of several compromise methods for rate compression should be adopted, depending primarily on concerns about administrability.

The Fairness of Community versus Experience Rating

Both sides of the community-rating debate attempt to preempt more detailed analysis by adopting competing fairness criteria. Employing the insurance industry's criterion of "actuarial fairness" makes it unfair *not* to rate according to individual risk, to the extent that it might constitute an unfair trade practice in many states to engage in community rating for conventional types of insurance (life, auto, and property, for example).[3] Philosopher Norman Daniels observes, however, that this risk-based fairness argument "confuses actuarial fairness with moral fairness."[4] Other theories of justice, such as Rawls's powerful argument, require society to care for the victims of nature's misfortunes. We are born with genetic defects, trapped in environmental influences we cannot change, and struck with random accidents and infectious illnesses. To say that we each have an individual right to ignore another person's unavoidable misery is a very thin fairness argument.

    A communitarian ethic holds that we should contribute equally toward sharing society's burdens.[5] Thus, community-rating advocates argue that a more social notion of fairness must prevail for health insurance, one that reflects the goal of universal coverage.[6] They suggest that only pure community rating captures the true soul of a socialized health insurance market, since only a single rate for each person spreads the risk of bad health evenly throughout society. However, the social characterization of insurance goes more to the criteria for eligibility than to the method of financing—that is, to who is covered, not how much they pay. Other social insurance systems employ a wide range of financing mechanisms, many of which are not community-rated in the same way proposed for health insurance.[7] The issue is not what form of financing best fits some a priori characterization of health insurance, but what form works best and is most socially responsible. The very concept of a single rate for each community acknowledges the validity of at least one risk-rating category—location. This allows substantial price variation—100 percent or more—simply based on the fortuity of where one lives, on account of the widely varying costs of care among the states and between rural and urban locations.

More relevant to the fairness issue are arguments that go to tax equity. Community-rating advocates maintain that it is fair to charge each person the same price for the same amount of coverage. It is obvious, though, that some purchasers will use this product much more than others and therefore will bear much greater responsibility for its cost. Therefore, the harshest attack on community rating in a market of mandatory purchase is that it creates a redistributive and hidden cross-subsidy from younger, healthier subscribers to older, sicker ones.[8] An unconstrained market allows a fivefold variation in individual insurance rates between young adults and near-retirees. Individuals who suffer from chronic illnesses such as diabetes and multiple sclerosis, or who have had bouts with cancer or heart disease, carry dramatically higher risks than their age-group averages. Requiring lower-risk subscribers to pay a higher premium than the market would charge to lower the costs for others can be seen as an implicit form of taxation or wealth transfer.

In New York, for instance, community rating was partially responsible for a 170 percent price increase by one large insurer for thirty-year-old males, and even a 30 percent increase for forty-five-year-old males.[9] David Bradford and Derrick Max roughly estimate that the Clinton plan would result in those aged twenty-five to thirty-four paying $26 billion more, and those aged fifty-five to sixty-four paying $33 billion less, as compared with an entirely age-adjusted rating system.[10] Henry Aaron and Barry Bosworth observe that adopting community rating will produce a greater redistribution than choosing whether government, business, or individuals will pay. Their rough calculations indicate that community rating will require employers in some industries to pay as much as $2,000 more and $4,000 less per employee than at present.[11] The Clinton administration calculates that community rating will require about 15 percent of families to pay somewhat more for insurance than they do now, and about 5 percent to pay as much as $500 a year more. These figures are for the individual portion of the premium only, and so do not reflect the employer's share.[12]

What disturbs critics about this cross-subsidy is not only its hidden nature but also its highly regressive incidence. Community-rated premiums, if viewed as a tax, amount to a head tax, which is considered one of the most regressive forms of taxation.[13] Moreover, since the cross-subsidy burden falls heaviest on younger workers, who tend to earn the lowest wages, community rating can be viewed as a perversely regressive form of taxation that subsidizes those who are better off. Feldman and Dowd, for instance, roughly estimated (using assumptions that do not necessarily apply to any pending proposal) that community rating would result in families headed by persons under twenty-five years old paying about twice their actuarial value, and families headed by persons fifty-five to sixty-four paying only three-quarters of their actuarial value. This subsidy of several thousand dollars per family would flow from a group that earns \$22,477 per year to one earning \$47,852 a year in 1991.[14]

These characterizations depend on two underlying assumptions, however, both of which are subject to challenge. First, they assume that individuals have a property right to trade on their individual risk status. It can be argued to the contrary that actuarially calculated insurance risk is not an innate personal endowment such as one's intelligence, physical strength, or beauty, which one can be said to have an inherent right to exploit. One's risk status is a statistical construct that is formed only to the extent that acquiring individual risk information produces a cost-effective market advantage. Market-derived health risk is so capricious that it changes simply according to the job one holds, the area where one lives, or the risk profile of others who happen to hold the same job or select the same insurer. Community rating can be characterized as an attempt to cure the market defects that are destroying the individual and small-group insurance market. This restructuring can be viewed as merely correcting the market-derived source of one's risk status rather than as a forced redistribution from those who have most benefited from the destructive effects of medical underwriting.

The second assumption made by some redistributive-subsidy critics is that the alternative to community rating is a fully risk-rated market. To the contrary, most individuals who will be required to contribute to a community rate under the Clinton plan already belong to a community-rated plan of sorts, one that sets a single rate for their employee group. Although group insurance is usually described as experience-rated, this is true only between groups. Within groups, a stricter version of community rating exists than even the Clinton plan requires, since many employers do not vary the employee's contribution according to the type of insurance chosen or according to as many categories of family status as are contained in the Clinton plan. Since the market is now generating many of the same types of cross-subsidies that community-rating opponents attack, their attack must be restricted only to that portion of the market that does not voluntarily engage in some form of group rating and that would not do so under market reforms.

I have pursued this line of argument a bit too far, however. Risk differentials are real. Therefore, the redistributive effect of the implicit wealth transfer cannot be imagined away, especially where participation in a community-rated system is mandatory. Nevertheless, another way to counter the regressive subsidy created by community rating is to view health risk over the span of each worker's lifetime rather than at a moment in time. Then it might be said that younger workers are not carrying an unfair burden, considering that they will receive the benefits of the subsidy themselves when they are older, much as those who contribute now to social security will be its recipients later.

This longitudinal perspective fails to rehabilitate community rating. If we ask ourselves what is a rational way to allocate the lifetime expenses of medical treatment to different portions of our productive careers, we would not likely favor an even burden over time; instead, we would more likely want a lower burden during the low-wage years and a higher burden later. Wages for males[15] increase approximately twofold over a career, tending to increase rapidly at the outset and to peak at around ages forty-five to fifty.[16] Male health risk varies three-to-four–fold between young and old workers, and it increases more rapidly in later years.[17] The parallels between average health risk and average asset accumulation are even stronger, since wealth (net worth) varies five-to-ten–fold on average across age groups and tends to increase rapidly during one's forties and fifties.[18] Therefore, the preferred distribution of health care costs over time would come much closer to some form of age-adjusted premiums than it would to pure community rating.[19] In particular, Senator Chafee's and Representative Cooper's proposals to limit age-adjustment to a twofold differential matches nicely with average, aggregate income growth.

I do not mean to paint too rosy a picture of risk rating—only to examine the various strands of analysis that shed light on the fairness issue. The lifetime distribution argument is only one such strand, which looks at an average person's preferred distribution of health care expenses over an earning career. This strand of analysis does not examine differential burdens across the income categories of different lifetime earners. That is, it ignores the fact that one earner (say, a banker) will have much less a burden than another (say, a bank teller) over their respective lifetime earnings. And this analysis is overly simplistic in assuming that health risk is homogenous for each age group. Still, this analysis shows that the fairness arguments are not so compelling on either side of the debate as to preempt consideration of the efficiency and feasibility of competing rating methods.

The Efficiency of Experience Rating

The efficiency argument that has the strongest force against community rating in a market of mandatory insurance purchase[20] is that charging everyone a single price will encourage free riding by those whose voluntary lifestyle behavior imposes costs on the insurance pool—behavior such as smoking, overeating, not wearing seat belts, not exercising, hang gliding, and engaging in unprotected sex.[21] This argument has dimensions of both efficiency and fairness. The efficiency argument holds that charging individuals according to voluntary health risks will encourage them to reduce risky behavior, thereby promoting the goal of prevention. The argument from fairness holds that even if individuals ignore price incentives, it violates standards of personal responsibility and moral blameworthiness to force those with conscientious health habits to pay for the costs created by voluntarily risky behavior. Both arguments are underscored by major themes in the Clinton reform campaign.

Community-rating proponents respond that many or most health risks are uncontrollable, and for these it would be neither fair nor efficient to impose their costs on individuals. The difficulty with this response is that health risk is clearly both controllable and uncontrollable to considerable degrees. One reads assertions that anywhere from 20 to 70 percent of health care costs are attributable to voluntary behavior,[22] but little rigorous empirical research backs up these claims. In part, this is because we lack any social consensus on what behavior is truly voluntary and what amounts to an illicit measure of social coercion. Genetic disease, for instance, is often cited as the quintessential uncontrollable health condition, but many conditions for which we are genetically predisposed such as cancer or heart disease are triggered to varying extents by controllable environmental influences such as smoking, diet, and lifestyle. Moreover, even for a highly deterministic genetic disease such as cystic fibrosis, extremists might argue that the child's parents should have to pay more because prenatal testing gives them the choice over whether to bring a defective newborn into existence. This callous argument highlights the fact that even perfectly controllable health risks may implicate privileged lifestyle habits that we would be loathe to penalize, even under a purely libertarian outlook. Should we pay more for not adhering to a strictly vegetarian diet? For driving long commutes to work?[23]

In addition to whether health risks are controllable, the efficiency argument depends on showing that people's unhealthy behavior is affected by price. If not, the fairness argument would still stand, but no actual reduction in health care costs would result from increased risk rating. Community-rating proponents argue that, if the threat of a debilitating illness or painful death is not sufficient to convince people to avoid bad health habits, a few extra dollars each month of insurance premiums certainly will not make a world of difference. Human psychology is not so one-dimensional, however, as to be reducible to such simplistic extrapolations. It may be that even modest financial incentives can have a stronger effect on some people's behavior than the risk of death, because money is a more immediate reward and the risk of death is a penalty that is subject to psychological denial.

In fact, several studies have demonstrated a rather strong association between individual costs and health habits. Cigarette smoking, for example, has been shown to have a price elasticity of demand of about -.5, which means that a 10 percent increase in the costs of cigarettes produces about a 5 percent reduction in smoking.[24] More anecdotally, one corporation that required its workers to pay $250 a year more for each of four specified risk factors (overweight, high cholesterol, high blood pressure, and smoking) saw health insurance claims for participants decline by 42 percent, while claims for nonparticipants rose 92 percent. The program also helped the employees to lose weight, lower their blood pressure, and quit smoking.[25]

Even if *individuals* do not respond strongly to risk-rated insurance, *employers* certainly do, and it is employers that have the largest stake in the cost of insurance. Largely because group insurance is now experienced-rated, many employers are instituting health promotion and wellness programs that are capable of having a major beneficial influence on employees' health. These programs include on-site exercise facilities, flu shots, and cancer screening. They also include targeted financial incentives to quit smoking, lose weight, improve diets, and the like. Most evaluations of these programs show them to be highly effective.[26] Experience-rated workers' compensation insurance has been shown to have the same positive influence on employers' work-place safety efforts.[27]

Under the Clinton plan, employers would lose any incentive to continue their health promotion efforts unless the company is large enough to opt out of the regional alliance system. Nonetheless, a fully risk-rated system penalizes employers and individuals for health risks they cannot control, and it prices insurance out of the reach of many people. The challenge is to devise a modified rating system that is capable of distinguishing the sheep from the goats.

One possibility, suggested by Mark Pauly, is a system of subsidies that compensates high-risk subscribers for uncontrollable or unaffordable risks, but this would be a hugely complex and expensive undertaking. Another possibility is to community rate the employee contribution but experience rate the employer's contribution. This is not easily compatible, however, with a managed competition system that fixes the employer's contribution according to a single reference plan. Therefore, it may be that these efficiency and fairness concerns can be better handled under a (partially or fully) community-rated system that employs targeted incentives to encourage health promotion. Senators Don Nickels and Phil Gramm, for instance, in separate bills propose credits to employers who maintain health promotion programs, just as some employers now reward their employees for exercising and not smoking. However, a system of administered incentives would require a new regulatory apparatus and a nonexistent methodology to do a job that is beginning to be done by the market.

A better compromise might be to community rate a set of basic benefits much leaner than those mandated by the Clinton plan, but to allow risk rating of supplemental insurance within rating bands.[28] Some degree of experience rating for supplemental insurance would preserve market-based health promotion incentives for those who choose to subscribe, while the community rating of the basic package would ensure an affordable decent minimum for those whose risk status or spending preferences preclude them from buying supplemental coverage.

The Feasibility of Community Rating

The host of fairness and efficiency arguments surveyed to this point has left us with the indeterminate result that neither side of the debate is wholly convincing. The rate compression accomplished by community rating helps to equalize the burden of medical costs and to keep insurance affordable for all, but it does so through an implicit and regressive subsidy. Relieving individuals and employers from the effects of their cost-increasing behavior creates irresponsible and inefficient incentives, but no simple risk-rating system accurately targets only controllable risks. This stalemate suggests that compromise forms of rating are plausible. It also suggests that more pragmatic concerns over administrability should carry the day in striking the optimal balance between risk pooling and risk segmenting. Therefore, I turn last to concerns over whether community rating is feasible.

It is sometimes said that community rating is essential to managed competition because it forces insurers to stop competing on the basis of how well they select risk.[29] Just the opposite is true. Community rating greatly intensifies insurers' incentives to engage in risk selection for the very reason that it precludes them from adjusting the premium to reflect individual risk. The need to control incentives for biased selection on the part of both insurers and subscribers creates formidable problems in administering a community-rated market.

The greatest concerns over feasibility exist in a voluntary market because there the low-risk subscribers who are asked to contribute the largest subsidies are able to opt out. This increases the average community rate even more, which drives out additional subscribers at the margin, thereby threatening to set off an adverse selection spiral that could destroy the market altogether or at least greatly increase the number of uninsured. As a result of these fears, virtually all health insurers except Blue Cross (which has no choice) pulled out of the market for individual purchase in New York when it was recently community-rated.[30]

These concerns are real for the portion of the Clinton plan that addresses supplemental insurance, most of which must also be community-rated.[31] The severe adverse selection that is likely to result has led some critics to charge that community rating is intended to make the market in supplemental insurance nonviable in order to produce a single-tier health care system. An adverse selection spiral is not a concern, however, for the basic benefits package, since no selection against the market can occur when purchase is mandatory. Nevertheless, community rating causes other forms of biased selection that raise a different set of problems relating to the uneven grouping of good and bad risks within the market.

Biased Selection among Insurers

In a market of mandatory purchase, community rating can produce two forms of biased selection among insurers: systemic and strategic. Systemic risk selection refers to naturally occurring unevenness in risk distribution. This can result either from insurers having different risk pools at the outset of community rating, or from random luck-of-the-draw as the community-rated market develops. These artificial price differences would level out over time if people who switched insurers were of equal risk with those who stayed. Then, insurers with lower risk pools would attract new subscribers who represent a cross section of the market. Existing good and bad risks would regress to the mean, and the deck would be partially reshuffled for those insurers who received a bad luck of the draw in the past. However, insurers fear for good reason that those who switch plans are systematically healthier than average, particularly when they join managed-care plans. This is because sicker patients are more attached to their existing doctors and therefore more reluctant to switch to obtain a price advantage.

As a consequence, insurers fear that companies with an initial artificial price advantage will be able to build on the advantage each year so that those who are only slightly behind at the outset will fall further behind each year. Eventually, the price disparity could become great enough to force some insurers out of business regardless of their inherent efficiency. Short of this extreme, this dynamic would result in what economists call dead-weight loss for the total market.

Even if historical and accidental risk differentials can be ironed out, a second form of biased selection will occur because of strategic behavior, by both insurers and subscribers. Many aspects of insurers' behavior toward their subscribers and attributes of their plans are differentially attractive to patients with different risk profiles. Therefore, insurers are able to engage in countless techniques that encourage enrollment by younger or healthier patients and disenrollment by older or sicker ones. Some risk, selection techniques are devious and improper, such as poor claims service for sicker patients, or locating the enrollment office on the top floor of a building without an elevator. Other techniques are innocuous. Well-baby visits and an ample supply of pediatric specialists attract younger subscribers, and specialists in sports medicine attract healthy subscribers. Choosing one advertising medium rather than another (fitness magazines versus *Modern Maturity*) or marketing more aggressively in one part of town rather than another is likely to produce widely varying combinations of age and health status.

Selection bias has been an ongoing, serious problem within the Federal Employees Health Benefits Program (FEHBP), which is the largest existing managed-competition network. Adverse selection resulted in the high-option (low deductible) fee-for-service plan in one area attracting risks that were 50 percent higher than the plan's actuarial value based on standard risks, whereas the low-option (high deductible) version of the same plan attracted risks that were about 40 percent lower than the plan's value based on standard risks.[32] Another study found that a different insurer, which offered two different plans with the same actuarial value, attracted FEHB subscribers with 79 percent higher claims to one plan than to the other.[33] As a consequence of these adverse selection problems, several fee-for-service plans and dozens of HMOs withdrew from FEHB during the late 1980s. Similar problems have plagued the California Public Employees Retirement System (CALPERS)[34] as well as large private employers offering multiple options. In one study of a private employer, a high-option plan attracted enrollees that were as much as four times more expensive than those who chose the low-option plan.[35] Finally, pronounced biased selection by Medicare enrollees between HMOs and traditional coverage has resulted in the federal government's losing rather than saving money on HMOs.[36] Most of these examples resulted more from patients' natural preferences for one type of coverage over another, rather than from insurers' purposeful manipulation of the market.

In sum, biased selection is likely to occur both naturally, through patients' choice among different kinds of insurance, and as a result of insurers' calculated use of covert selection devices. Premiums therefore will not perfectly reflect each insurer's inherent efficiency in the administration of insurance or the management of care. Competitive advantages gained by cost savings or service quality will be negated by these distorting effects on price, which will undermine one of the purposes of a market-based system. The opportunities for systemic-selection bias increase the more that choice is exercised on an individual (as opposed to group) basis, and the opportunities for covert risk-selection strategies increase as health insurance moves toward managed care. Under the pure indemnity model with free choice of physician, insurance policies could be made more or less attractive only by varying their benefits. With managed care, the attractiveness of plans varies across a much wider spectrum determined by the style of medical practice and the structure of the treatment network.

A number of these techniques can be controlled, but it is neither possible nor desirable to police all avenues and motivations for selection. Demand-side selection, for instance, could be reduced by changing open enrollment to every three years or by requiring each work force to join a single plan as a group, but these remedies have obvious consequences for consumer choice. The inevitable path of this regulatory approach is to stamp out almost all forms of variety, to make a competitive process workable.

There are two alternative remedies. The first would abandon or modify community rating, while the second would provide some behind-the-scenes adjustment. Allowing competing insurers some variation in their premiums to reflect relative risks among different pools of patients combats biased selection by requiring subscribers to pay more of the actuarial value of their individual health risks. More accurate risk rating tends to make both good and bad risks equally attractive to every insurer in a competitive market, thereby counteracting insurers' incentive to encourage favorable selection.

The other remedy is to adopt a system of risk adjustment, which accomplishes the same result without passing risk differences on to individual consumers. If risk adjustment works well, insurers receive accurate compensation for individual risks and therefore have no distorting incentives to attract better risks or discourage worse ones. This forces them to compete on the basis of the efficiency-enhancing attributes of their plans. And if risk adjustment works well, premium differentials can be compressed or strict community rating enforced without unfair burden to high-risk subscribers and their insurers. Risk adjustment is therefore the *deus ex machina* of community rating—the solution to all our problems that magically descends from above. Only one problem remains: does it work?

Techniques for Risk Adjustment

The Clinton reform proposal is conspicuously silent on techniques for risk adjustment, leaving this black box to be opened by future regulators. The same is true for every other major proposal for managed competition, including those by the Jackson Hole Group and the earlier proposal by the Bush administration. Each of these proposals delegates the judgment of what the appropriate risk adjustment technique should be to expert determination. This deference to experts carries an implicit message of hopeful optimism: plenty of proven risk adjusters are in use, and it is merely a technical matter to determine which is the best. In truth, this is hardly an accurate portrayal of the state of the art in risk adjustment. Several adjusters have been developed, but they are all early in their testing and refinement processes, and each is plagued with considerable flaws.

Demographic factors such as age, sex, and occupation are the risk-measurement tools in widest use by the insurance industry and the government. They explain only a small percentage, however, of the total variation in individual health care costs. For instance, the adjusted average per capita cost (AAPCC) method that HCFA uses to pay Medicare HMOs accounts for less than 1 percent of the variation in costs of treatment among individual Medicare beneficiaries.[37] Attempts to improve these demographic measures by including the individual's earlier use of health care resources have had only modest success, increasing the explanation of variance to around 2 percent.[38]

Measures of actual health condition can be expected to perform considerably better depending on their sophistication, but the more sophisticated measures create additional difficulties. One is the problem of collecting sufficient and accurate information. How far back do we look at health status, and to what sources? Some health-condition risk adjusters rely on episodes of inpatient hospitalization collected from claims data. Claims data are notoriously skimpy, however, on actual clinical information, and they may not exist at all within staff- and group-model HMOs. Better information can be garnered from medical records, but these are not computerized or systematized. Also, using medical records raises sensitive issues of confidentiality, particularly in the context of an employment-based insurance system that might give employers access to personal information. Moreover, a system based on past treatment leaves out entirely anyone who has not been hospitalized in the relevant time frame. One attempt to correct the latter flaw relies on outpatient treatment encounters, but then the data collection problems are greatly amplified.

Health status measures for risk adjustment also create several problems of bias and distortion, depending on the particular measure used. Consider, for instance, a measure that relies on recent past medical treatment. This would encourage insurers to call in all subscribers for treatment just before measurement time. Consider instead a measure that looks at the patient's actual condition, as indicated by diagnoses. As we know from the Medicare prospective payment system, diagnoses can also be manipulated. Moreover, adjusting for health status creates a perverse reward for plans that provide inferior treatment. Similar concerns relate to treatment efficiency. If a health status adjustment measure uses past treatment, and even if this measure is not manipulated, it still has the effect of rewarding those plans that overtreat and penalizing those that are more economical. These two flaws undermine the ability of a competitive market system to reward efficiency in the management of health care.[39]

The developers of health status measures for risk adjustment are conscious of these problems, and so they design their measures to avoid them. They search for the most easily accessible and reliable sources of data, and they restrict their inquiry to diagnoses and items of treatment that are less subject to discretionary judgment or manipulation. In doing so, however, they must necessarily sacrifice some degree of accuracy by forgoing valuable information. As a consequence, these measures have shown only limited success. The most sophisticated measures still predict less than 10 percent of the variation among individual health care costs over the course of a year.[40]

Nevertheless, this effort is certainly worth pursuing if usable health risk adjusters might emerge. That prospect hinges on how much of the variation in health care costs must be explained. The 5 to 8 percent explanation of variation currently achieved by health status measures may seem minuscule in the abstract, but not when one compares the figure with the percentage of total possible explainable variation. This perception also changes when we examine the degree of variation explainable at the level of a large group rather than at an individual level. These two points require additional discussion.

Perfect risk adjustment would be tantamount to cost-based reimbursement, since it would pay insurers exactly what it cost to treat each subscriber. Therefore, it is unrealistic to ask what percentage of *total* variation health adjustment measures explain; rather, we should judge them according to the portion of *explainable* variation they can explain. It is difficult to establish how much of the individual variation in health care costs can theoretically be predicted, but the few rough estimates that have been made suggest that explainable variation in individual health care costs ranges only from 15 to 20 percent. The rest of variation arises from true randomness.[41] Viewed in this light, the range of 5 to 8 percent that has already been achieved looks much better.

Moreover, variation of any sort, health care costs included, is much wider and much less subject to explanation (statistical prediction) at an individual than at a group level. Therefore, the percentage of variation explained increases dramatically when these risk adjustment measures are applied to group variation—that is, differences in costs between groups rather than among individuals within a group. Depending on the size of groups (from 50 to more than 1,000), the variation explained increases to well over 50 percent for the various risk adjusters that have been tested.[42]

The critical question for risk adjusters then becomes, Which test—individual or group prediction—is the appropriate one? The answer depends on refining our sense of why risk adjustment is important. One goal of risk adjustment is to level the uneven distribution of risks among competing insurers, so that their community-rated premiums more nearly reflect their comparative efficiencies in managing care and administering the insurance function. For this goal to be achieved, it is necessary only to predict risk at the level of the total risk pool. A second purpose of risk adjustment, however, is to remove insurers' incentive to engage in risk selection. Making good and bad risks equally attractive to insurers forces them to compete for business based on the attractiveness of their product rather than on their skills at risk selection. This purpose is advanced only if accurate risk prediction exists at the level at which insurers will solicit business.

Both the Clinton plan and the competing proposals for managed competition require insurers to compete for business at a retail rather than a wholesale level—that is, to market to individuals rather than to employer groups. Therefore, risk selection must be accurate at an individual level if it is to counteract incentives for risk selection.

But how accurate? Since the purpose is to counteract insurers' own risk-selection incentives, perfect risk prediction is not necessary. A risk adjuster need be only as accurate as insurers themselves at risk selection. In the past, insurers have relied on imprecise measures such as claims experience or demographics, so the task at hand seems all too easy. Mark Pauly argues, for instance, that a risk adjuster need only detect the 5 to 15 percent of applicants that insurers typically turn down for coverage or to whom they offer substandard rates.[43] However, this indicates only the level of overt risk selection in a fully risk-rated market. Community rating and the prohibition of direct medical underwriting will intensify the incentives to engage in more covert selection.

Even if academic researchers are convinced that they can explain as much or more individual variation as insurers, risk adjusters will not accomplish their goal unless insurance underwriters are convinced. Since underwriters rely on a variety of both subjective and objective risk indicators, including pure intuition—indicators that are not the same as the risk-adjustment measure—underwriters are likely to continue to believe, even if untrue, that it is possible to institute some system of risk adjustment. As Deborah Stone has observed, the techniques of risk assessment and underwriting "are so deeply embedded in the structure and mentality of insurance employees that they will be hard to eradicate. . . . Billions of dollars, millions of jobs, and innumerable organizations depend on the underwriting function," which will continue to exist in any event by virtue of the life and disability insurance business that most large health insurers also maintain.[44]

This does not mean that sufficient prediction of individual variation is not achievable—only that the task will require additional effort and continual vigilance. Confidence in risk adjustment will come only from real-world experience.

Retrospective Risk Adjustment and Reinsurance

A final salvation for the accuracy of risk adjustment is to conduct it on a retrospective rather than a prospective basis. This amounts to a form of reinsurance. Retrospective risk adjustment continuously monitors the actual costs of patient treatment—the very thing that prospective adjustment attempts to predict—and it varies premium payments accordingly. One component of New York's risk adjustment system, for instance, is to pay insurers a scheduled amount for each subscriber who receives treatment from a list of high-cost conditions such as AIDS or cancer. This amounts to a stop-loss form of reinsurance, because it shifts the insurance function for the listed costs from the individual insurer to the central risk-transfer pool.

Applied to discrete categories of cases, retrospective risk adjustment can be a useful backstop for the worst failings of prospective risk-adjustment measures, much as outlier payments under Medicare DRGs correct for that system's largest inaccuracies. If applied across-the-board, however, this form of adjustment would render the insurance function meaningless, since insurers would then bear no risk for any of their costs. Naturally, this is not proposed, but it demonstrates the inherent danger in retrospective adjusters—namely, that they remove from the insurer the incentive to control the costs of care. They do so for the very cases where costs are the highest, and hence control may be the most important. This also places insurance risk on the entity that funds the transfer pool. If this is the health alliance, one of the fundamental limitations on the alliance's authority is contradicted. Risk-bearing health alliances are tantamount to a single-payer system. Therefore, truly retrospective risk adjusters should be used sparingly and in a manner that retains some incentive for cost control.[45]

Another alternative to mandatory risk adjustment is the voluntary reinsurance mechanism employed in small-group market reforms that have been adopted in a number of states.[46] These voluntary reinsurance pools adjust for uneven distribution of risk and neutralize the incentive to select against bad risks by allowing insurers to pass their high-risk groups and individuals on to a central market pool. The advantage of voluntary reinsurance[47] over an administered risk-adjustment system is that reinsurance allows insurers to decide for themselves which are the high-risk cases. Academic researchers and government administrators, therefore, need not outguess the industry's underwriters. In addition, since the predictable losses by the reinsured pool are made up by assessments (usually against insurers themselves), reinsurance makes more explicit the internal subsidies built into a community-rated system.[48]

This form of risk adjustment is not a perfect one, however, because the reinsurance decision itself requires skill in risk selection and so would still reward insurers for their selection abilities. Moreover, reinsurance is particularly unsuited in the context of community rating, because it applies only to *high*-risk cases; it does not neutralize the incentive to attract lower risks.

Reinsurance works better under a rating band system that allows some flexibility in risk rating. Community rating allows insurers to profit from low-risk cases, whereas in a pricing system that allows some rate variation, market forces will drive premium prices down for low-risk subscribers. Therefore, risk adjustment is not necessary at the low end of the range unless low risks fall below the rating bands. However, lower rates tend naturally to stay within a reasonable range of the market average, because no person is so healthy as to be many times less likely than average to have no expenses. Put another way, enough people are healthy that no one stands out as *extremely* healthy.[49] The same is not true for unhealthy people. Their insurance risks are so high they will far exceed the rating bands. Consequently, a reinsurance mechanism is necessary to distribute fairly the resulting burden of taking on high-risk subscribers. In short, although a reinsurance mechanism does not fit well with community rating, its use in a market that allows some variation in rates may be a sensible alternative to the administrative problems created by regulatory risk adjustment.

Conclusion

When I began this project, I promised myself to refrain from prescribing solutions to the community-rating dilemma. It would be unsatisfying, however, to finish this analysis without drawing at least the following conclusions:

First, the internal logic of private health insurance markets must be respected in any attempt to harness market forces to achieve social objectives. Private insurers should not be given a role they are inherently incapable of assuming, nor should the benefits of a private market mechanism be sapped in the process of market reform. Primarily, this requires that some degree of risk rating be retained. Risk assessment is fundamental to the functioning of private insurance, and it provides social benefits by creating incentives for risk reduction. Controlling the excesses of risk rating does not require its elimination altogether.

Of course, it is plausible to allow some form of cross-subsidization to exist in the manner by which private health insurance is priced. Insurers must recognize the larger social function that health insurance has assumed as the primary vehicle for financing the costs of universal health care access. More explicit forms of subsidization than rate compression and guaranteed issue might be conceivable and even desirable, but government has rarely succeeded in crafting an unobjectionable redistributive program.

Second, because of adverse selection, pure community rating creates severe feasibility problems in a market of voluntary purchase, particularly for individual insurance and very small groups. Community rating can function in a market of mandatory purchase, but biased selection among insurers usually creates pricing distortions that undermine the purpose of a market mechanism and that may unfairly drive some insurance companies entirely out of business. Therefore, a workable risk-adjustment mechanism is an essential adjunct to community rating. The problem is that such mechanisms are still new and relatively undeveloped, and hence are plagued with problems of accuracy, distortion, and administrability. One pragmatic compromise to consider while risk-adjustment methods are being further refined would be to allow a degree of risk variation similar to that permitted by the rating bands contained in industry-sponsored small-group market reforms, coupled with a voluntary reinsurance mechanism. Other compromise positions may also be viable, such as risk adjusting a much leaner set of community-rated basic benefits and encouraging a much more active market in risk-rated supplemental insurance.[50]

Notes

1. Several prominent health economists are opposed, however. See, for example, Roger Feldman and Bryan E. Dowd, "Biased Selection—Fairness and Efficiency in Health Insurance Markets," in Robert B. Helms, ed., *American Health Policy: Critical Issues for Reform* (Washington, D.C.: AEI Press, 1993), pp. 64–86; Mark Pauly, "Killing with Kindness: Why Some Forms of Managed Competition Might Needlessly Stifle Competitive Managed Care," conference paper presented at American Enterprise Institute's conference, Health Care Expenditure Controls: Political and Economic Issues, April 21–22, 1993.

2. For a detailed discussion, see Mark A. Hall, *Reforming Private Health Insurance* (Washington, D.C.: AEI Press, forthcoming 1994).

3. See generally, Kenneth S. Abraham, "Efficiency and Fairness in Insurance Risk Classification," *Virginia Law Review*, vol. 71 (1985), pp. 403–51.

4. Norman Daniels, "Insurability and the HIV Epidemic: Ethical Issues in Underwriting," *Milbank Quarterly*, vol. 68, no. 4 (1990), pp. 497–525.

5. Discussing the application of communitarian principles, see generally, Mark A. Hall, "Community Rating or Experience Rating?" *The Responsive Community*, vol. 2, no. 4 (Fall 1992), pp. 79–82.

6. Deborah Stone, "The Struggle for the Soul of Health Insurance," *Journal of Health Politics, Policy and Law*, vol. 18, no. 2 (Summer 1993), pp. 286–317; Norman Daniels, "Insurability and the HIV Epidemic: Ethical Issues in Underwriting," *Milbank Quarterly*, vol. 68, no. 4 (1990), pp. 497–525; Donald W. Light, "The Practice and Ethics of Risk-Rated Health Insurance," *Journal of the American Medical Association*, vol. 267, no. 18 (1992), pp. 2503–08.

7. For instance, unemployment insurance premiums, which are a percentage of payroll, are roughly proportionate to the risk insured, whereas Medicaid funding is a progressive and broad-based tax. Thomas Bodenheimer and Kevin Grumbach, "Financing Universal Health Insurance: Taxes, Premiums, and the Lessons of Social Insurance," *Journal of Health Politics, Policy and Law*, vol. 17, no. 3 (Fall 1992), pp. 439–62.

8. In addition, the Clinton proposal requires rural areas to subsidize urban areas depending on how alliance boundaries are drawn. It also creates a cross-subsidy between two-career and one-career families by requiring employers of each worker to contribute the same amount regardless of whether the worker's spouse is also employed. In brief, the complex methodology results in two-worker families contributing 70 percent more than one-worker families if the average number of workers per family is 1.5. These subsidy effects raise different social policies than the ones I explore here.

9. Henry Gilgoff, "Dialing in Desperation: Coming Change in Insurance Law Sparks Panic," *Newsday,* March 12, 1993. However, these increases also reflect underlying increases in the cost of care. For group insurance, projections by Blue Cross, Aetna, and the American Academy of Actuaries based on existing business indicate that about 10 percent of small groups (fewer than twenty-five employees) would experience price increases of 40 percent or more, and about 20 percent of groups would have increases of 20 percent or more if the small-group market were community-rated. American Academy of Actuaries, "An Analysis of Mandated Community Rating," March 1993; William R. Jones, Charles T. Doe, and Jonathan M. Topodas, "Pure Community Rating: A Quick Fix to Avoid," *Journal of American Health Policy,* Jan./Feb. 1993, pp. 29–33 (representing AETNA). A different simulation estimated that 12 to 33 percent of the premium for subscribers with actuarial costs below the average community rate goes to subsidize subscribers with above-average risks. Roger L. Pupp, "Community Rating and Cross Subsidies in Health Insurance," *Journal of Risk and Insurance,* vol. 48 (Dec. 1981), pp. 610–27. By contrast, the American Academy of Actuaries estimates that adjusting community rating for age would produce increases of more than 20, and 40 percent for only 4 and 2 percent, respectively, of the existing individual and small-group market.

10. David F. Bradford and Derrick Max, "Community Rating in Clinton's Health Reform: Another Hit to the Young?" American Enterprise Institute working paper, Nov. 16, 1993 draft. These numbers attribute the entire premium to individuals rather than deducting the employer share, under the assumption that employer contributions lower take-home pay.

11. Henry J. Aaron and Barry Bosworth, "Economic Issues in Reform of Health Care Financing," The Brookings Institution (1993). They are corroborated by Lewin-VHI, which estimates that community rating would save 16 percent of businesses $2,500 or more per employee, and would cost 21 percent of businesses $1,000 or more per employee. However, those who would have to pay more include many businesses that now offer no insurance. *Business and Health,* (Jan. 1994), p. 12. Lewin-VHI also estimates that the community rate for employers is increased 14 percent by adding nonworkers to the pool.

12. Editorial, "A Misleading Health Estimate," *New York Times,* Nov. 3, 1993, p. A14.

13. Observe that this only holds true for the employee's or individual's portion of the premium. For the employer, the regressive feature depends on whether the premium is thought to come out of the employer's profits or from the employees' wages.

14. Roger Feldman and Bryan E. Dowd, "Biased Selection—Fairness and Efficiency in Health Insurance Markets," in Helms, *American Health Policy,* pp. 64–86.

15. I focus on males because they are more likely to have an uninterrupted career and because they are frequently the principal wage-earners whose employers provide dependent coverage. For females, changes in both wages and health risk are flatter.

16. Bruce E. Kaufman, *The Economics of Labor Markets,* 3rd. ed (Fort Worth: Dryden Press), p. 335; Kevin M. Murphy and Finis Welch, "Empirical Age-Earnings Profiles," *Journal of Labor Economics,* vol. 8, no. 2 (April 1990), pp. 202–29.

17. U.S. Government Accounting Office, "Employer-Based Health Insurance: High Costs, Wide Variation Threaten System," Sept. 1992, p. 32.

18. U.S. Department of Commerce, *Household Wealth and Asset Ownership: 1988*, Survey of Income and Program Participation, Series P-70, no. 22; Arthur Kennickell and Janice Shack-Marquez. "Changes in Family Finances from 1983 to 1989: Evidence from the Survey of Consumer Finances," *Federal Reserve Bulletin*, Jan. 1992, pp. 1–18.

19. For similar reasons, social policies that protect the elderly and burden the young are increasingly coming under attack as the aging of the baby boom generation threatens to bankrupt funding mechanisms for Social Security and Medicare. See generally, P. Johnson, C. Conrad, and D. Thompson, eds., *Workers versus Pensioners: Intergenerational Justice in an Aging World* (New York: St. Martin's Press, 1989); H.J. Aaron, B.P. Bosworth, and G. Burless, *Can America Afford to Grow Old?* (Washington, D.C.: The Brookings Institution, 1989); Phillip Longman, *Born to Pay: The New Politics of Aging in America* (Boston: Houghton-Mifflin, 1987).

20. Other attacks are primarily relevant to a market of voluntary purchase. See Roger Feldman and Bryan E. Dowd, "Biased Selection—Fairness and Efficiency in Health Insurance Markets," in Helms, *American Health Policy*, pp. 64–86; Mark V. Pauly, "The Welfare Economics of Community Rating," *Journal of Risk and Insurance*, vol. 37 (Sept. 1970), pp. 407–18.

21. The evidence is clear that bad health habits increase health insurance premiums, even if they do not necessarily increase total social costs. James Fries, C. Everett Koop, Carson E. Beadle, et al., "Reducing Health Care Costs by Reducing the Need and Demand for Medical Services," *New England Journal of Medicine*, vol. 329 (1993), pp. 321–25 (people with bad health habits have annual claims costs eight times higher than those with good health habits); W. G. Manning, E.B. Keeler, J.P. Newhouse, et al., *The Costs of Poor Health Habits* (Cambridge, Mass: Harvard Univ. Press, 1991).

22. Fries, Koop, Beadle, et al., "Reducing Health Care Costs."; R. William Whitmer, "Why We Should Foster Health Promotion," *Business and Health*, Nov. 1993, p. 68. See also J. Michael McGinnis and William H. Foege, "Actual Causes of Death in the United States," *JAMA*, vol. 270 (1993), pp. 2207–12 (the leading causes of death result from preventable behavior such as smoking, diet, and drinking).

23. For a forceful expression of these concerns, see Robert L. Schwartz, "Making Patients Pay for Their Lifestyle Choices," *Cambridge Quarterly of Healthcare Ethics*, vol. 4 (1992), pp. 393–400.

24. Theodore E. Keeler, Teh-Wei Hu, Paul G. Barnett, and Willard G. Manning, "Taxation, Regulation, and Addiction: A Demand Function for Cigarettes Based on Time-Series Evidence," *Journal of Health Economics*, vol. 12 (1993), pp. 1–18.

25. BNA Health Care Daily, July 8, 1993. See generally, K. Pelletier. "A Review and Analysis of the Health and Cost-Effective Outcome Studies of Comprehensive Health Promotion and Disease Prevention Programs.," *American Journal of Health Promotion*, vol. 5 (1991), p. 311–15.

26. Fries, Koop, Beadle, et al., "Reducing Health Care Costs."; Regina E. Herzlinger and David Calkins, "How Companies Tackle Health Care Costs: Part III," *Harvard Business Review*, Jan./Feb. 1986, pp. 70–79.

27. Christopher J. Bruce and Frank J. Atkins, "Efficiency Effects of Premium-setting Regimes under Worker's Compensation: Canada and the United States," *Journal of Labor Economics*, vol. 11 (1993), pp. S38–S67 (a change from community to experience

rating reduced the fatality rate by 40 percent in forestry and 20 percent in construction); M. Moore and W.K. Viscusi, *Compensation Mechanisms for Job Risks: Wages, Workers' Compensation, and Product Liability* (Princeton: Princeton University Press, 1990) (workers' compensation in general reduces fatality rates 27 percent); John W. Ruser, "Workers' Compensation Insurance, Experience-Rating, and Occupational Injuries," *Rand Journal of Economics,* vol. 16 (1985), pp. 487–503.

28. This is analogous to the market structure for Medi-Gap coverage, which most Medicare recipients purchase to supplement Medicare coverage, except that Medi-Gap typically is age-adjusted community-rated.

One important complication of relying much more extensively on supplemental insurance is that supplemental insurance increases the cost of primary insurance because of the demand creation (moral hazard) effect of lowering copayments and deductibles. Another complication is that coordinating between two separate insurers is much more difficult in a managed care environment than under a pure indemnity model. The Clinton plan resolves these problems by requiring purchasers of supplemental cost-sharing policies to buy only from the primary health plan. Another alternative is to require supplemental insurers to make a risk-adjustment payment to the primary insurer, but to allow the primary insurer to control the delivery network.

29. See, for example, "A Misleading Health Estimate," editorial, *New York Times,* Nov. 3, 1993.

30. The adverse selection effects are not as strong for group purchasers, so that portion of the market still remains viable. For additional discussion, see Hall, *Reforming Private Health Insurance.*

31. The Health Security Act requires cost-sharing supplemental policies to be community-rated (H.R. 3600, sec. 1423(c)(1)), but it is silent on the rating of policies that cover benefits not offered in the basic plan. Because the basic plan is so comprehensive, it is likely the cost-sharing supplement will be the more important one.

32. Although the risk-neutral value of the high-option plan was only 42 percent greater than the low-option plan, the actual costs (measured by experience-based premiums charged) for subscribers in the high-option plan were 264 percent higher. Institute of Medicine, *Employment and Health Benefits: A Connection at Risk,* Marilyn J. Field and Harold T. Shapiro, eds. (Washington, D.C.: National Academy Press, 1993), p. 176.

33. Ibid. See also, M. Susan Marquis, "Adverse Selection with a Multiple Choice among Health Insurance Plans: A Simulation Analysis," *Journal of Health Economics,* vol. 11 (1992), pp. 129–51.

34. Harold Luft, et al., "Adverse Selection in a Large Multiple-Option Health Benefits Program," *Advances in Health Economics and Health Services Research,* in R. Scheffler and L. Rossiter, eds., vol. 6 (Greenwich, Conn.: JAI Press 1985), pp. 197–229.

35. R.P. Ellis, "The Effect of Prior-Year Health Expenditures on Health Coverage Plan Choice," in ibid.

36. Robert Pear, "Medicare to Stop Pushing Patients to Enter H.M.O.'s," *New York Times,* Dec. 27, 1993. See also, Joseph P. Newhouse, "Patients at Risk: Health Reform and Risk Adjustment," forthcoming 1994 (Medicare HMO enrollees used about 25 percent fewer resources than non-HMO enrollees).

37. Gerard F. Anderson, Earl P. Steinberg, Neil R. Powe, et al., "Setting Payment

Rates for Capitated Systems: A Comparison of Various Alternatives," *Inquiry*, vol. 27 (Fall 1990), pp. 225–33.

38. Mark C. Hornbrook, Michael L. Goodman, and Marjorie D. Bennett, "Assessing Health Plan Case Mix in Employed Populations: Ambulatory Morbidity and Prescribed Drug Models," in Mark C. Hornbrook, ed., *Advances in Health Economics and Health Services Research: Risk-Based Contributions to Private Health Insurance*, vol. 12 (Greenwich, Conn.: JAI Press, 1991), pp. 197–232.

39. Additional problems of bias and administrability arise from the manner in which a health risk measure is developed and tested and from the need to calibrate it to local communities and different types of insurance. See generally sources cited in the next note.

40. The literature is summarized and discussed in White House Task Force on Health Risk Pooling, *Health Risk Pooling for Small-Group Health Insurance* (January 1993); Anderson, Steinberg, Powe, et al., "Setting Payment Rates for Capitated Systems"; and Mark C. Hornbrook and Michael J. Goodman, "Health Plan Case Mix: Definition, Measurement, and Use," in Hornbrook, *Advances in Health Economics and Health Services Research*.

41. See J. Newhouse, W.G. Manning, E.B. Keeler, and E.M. Sloss, "Adjusting Capitation Rates Using Objective Health Measures and Prior Utilization," *Health Care Financing Review*, vol. 10, no. 3 (Spring 1989), pp. 41–53; Joseph P. Newhouse, "Patients at Risk: Health Reform and Risk Adjustment," forthcoming 1994.

42. See Stephen T. Hayes, "Demographic Risk Factors Derived from HMO Data," in Hornbrook, *Advances in Health Economics and Health Services Research*.

43. Mark Pauly, "Killing with Kindness: Why Some Forms of Managed Competition Might Needlessly Stifle Competitive Managed Care," conference paper presented at American Enterprise Institute, "Health Care Expenditure Controls: Political and Economic Issues," April 21–22, 1993.

44. Deborah Stone, "The Struggle for the Soul of Health Insurance," *Journal of Health Politics, Policy and Law*, vol. 18, no. 2 (Summer 1993), pp. 313.

45. Joseph Newhouse, for example, proposes a partial capitation rate that blends capitation with fee-for-service or cost-based reimbursement. Joseph P. Newhouse, "Patients at Risk: Health Reform and Risk Adjustment," forthcoming 1994. By adjusting the blend, a proper mix between cost-containing and risk-accepting incentives can be maintained across the spectrum of treatment costs.

46. For a more extensive discussion than the present space allows, see Hall, *Reforming Private Health Insurance*.

47. This form of reinsurance is voluntary in the sense that the decision to reinsure each group or individual is made by the insurer. It is mandatory, however, to the extent that all insurers must participate in funding the reinsurance pool.

48. Eugene Steuerle makes this point in "Community Rating of Health: How Much is Appropriate?" *Tax Notes*, May 31, 1993, p. 1269.

49. M. Berk and Alan Monheit, "The Concentration of Health Care Expenditures: An Update," *Health Affairs*, Winter 1992, pp. 145–49 (national figures, based on NMES 1987 data).

50. See text at note 28 above.

About the Author

MARK A. HALL is professor of law and public health at Wake Forest University School of Law and Bowman Gray School of Medicine. He is also an associate in management at the Babcock School of Management, all of which are located in Winston-Salem, North Carolina. Professor Hall has also completed a Robert Wood Johnson Foundation Health Finance Fellowship at Johns Hopkins University. He specializes in health care law and public policy, with a focus on economic, regulatory, and corporate issues. His present research interests include competition, integrated delivery systems, and insurance market reform.

AEI Studies in Health Policy

Special Studies in Health Reform

Other AEI Books on Health Policy